Abo the /

William Webb spent ten years as a radar technician in the RAF before becoming an ICAO listed expert in communications and navigation Aids.

He spent more than forty years travelling the world before using his experience to write his first three books.

His latest book, *The Best Medicine*, was inspired by the gift of an autograph book of a WW1 voluntary nurse.

Previous books;

        Non fiction:
        Been There, Done That, Got the T-Shirt
        My Art Is Where the Ohm Is

        Fiction:
        Per Ardua Ad Ulcers

Dedications

To my late dear friend Colin Hornsby without whose generosity this book would never have been published.

Also, to the many servicemen and nursing staff of World War One whose names have been long forgotten but whose sacrifices will ever be remembered.

William Webb

THE BEST MEDICINE

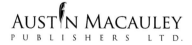
AUSTIN MACAULEY
PUBLISHERS LTD.

A CIP catalogue record for this title is available from the British Library.

ISBN 978 1 78455 245 9

www.austinmacauley.com

First Published (2014)
Austin Macauley Publishers Ltd.
25 Canada Square
Canary Wharf
London
E14 5LB

Printed and bound in Great Britain

Frontispiece

THE "BEST" MEDICINE

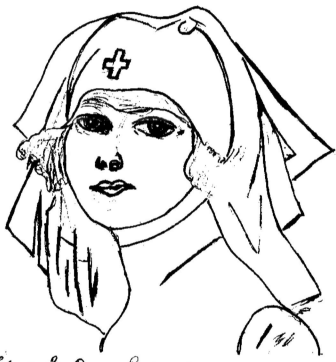

Pte Fr. Clark 2/4 Devon Regt 291614
With Best Wishes to Nurse Goodban
V.A.H. Barnstaple   Oct 23rd 1917

Ward II

Private Fr. Clark 291614
2/4 Devonshire Regiment
With Best Wishes to Nurse Goodban
VAH Barnstaple   Oct 23rd 1917

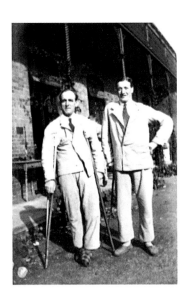

Private Clark, Devon Regt, and Trooper Venables, Inniskillen Dragoons

Foreword

Frances Josephine Hamlyn Goodban served as a volunteer (VAD) nurse with the British Red Cross from October 1914 until the 31st January 1919. She worked a total of 11,276 hours, largely in North Devon, for no pay at all. However, she did receive £15 in expenses for her nine months spent at the British Red Cross Hospital Netley, near Southampton, which probably did not even cover her travelling costs.

By coincidence, Agatha Christie also joined the Red Cross as a volunteer nurse in Devon in October 1914. However, she later qualified as a dispenser of medicine where she no doubt acquired her knowledge of poison which featured in many of her mystery novels. In contrast to Nurse Goodban, Agatha Christie only worked a total of 3,400 hours.

For the duration of the war Nurse Goodban worked at various VAD and British Red Cross hospitals. Specifically, these were Ilfracombe's Westwell Hospital (October 14th 1914 until March 15th 1915, and October 1918 until January 31st 1919) and Barnstaple VAD Hospitals (1915/1916 and 1917/1918). She also worked at the Red Cross Hospital at Netley in Hampshire in 1916/1917 and March 1918 until July 1918. Her tours of duty at Netley were no doubt precipitated by increased action, and therefore an increase in casualties, by the allied forces in Europe and Asia. During her years of service she tended hundreds of wounded servicemen from the British and Commonwealth forces that had been evacuated from the conflict.

Frances Goodban was born in the Lewisham district of London in 1878 to well-to-do parents. Her father, Joseph, was a deputy principle in the Bank of England and was born in Pimlico, London. Her mother, Anne Frances, was born in Ashford, North Devon. It was her second marriage, her first husband having died. By 1911 the family had moved to North Devon following Joseph's retirement.

Frances was 37 years of age and still unmarried when she decided to join the Voluntary Aid Detachment and become a volunteer nurse. The VAD was a scheme brought about by the War Office on the 16th August 1909. At the conclusion of the Boer War the Government was concerned that the existing medical and nursing services would not be enough to cope with the number of casualties in the event of any new hostilities. What with the evolution of new and improved guns, tanks, aircraft, and gas warfare they had good reason to be apprehensive.

Male and female Voluntary Aid Detachments were set up throughout England and Wales in 1909 with a similar scheme commencing in Scotland in December of the same year. By the time of the outbreak of war in 1914 there were 519 male detachments and 1757 female detachments registered with the War Office.

The female detachments mainly consisted of a Commandant, a Medical Officer, a Quartermaster, and twenty two women. Of this twenty two, at least two were trained nurses. Originally, the detachments were scheduled to meet at least once a month but most met weekly with the participants working towards gaining certificates in Home Nursing and First Aid. In some areas the volunteers were allowed to spend time in local civilian hospitals to gain experience in caring for the sick. The detachments were originally intended to staff auxiliary hospitals and rest stations in the UK. However, by the middle of 1915, VAD members were being shipped overseas to augment the number of trained nurses in military hospitals. Only VAD nurses aged 19 – 30 were considered for overseas duty, whereas those from 21 – 48 were eligible to work in the UK; which included Nurse Goodban.

On the commencement of the war Red Cross and Auxiliary Hospitals sprung up all over the UK. Public buildings, church halls, hotels, and even large private houses were commandeered and utilised to accommodate the thousands of casualties being shipped back to Britain. The proportion of trained nurses in these establishments was very small so VADs were called upon to carry out the bulk of the work. In addition to mundane tasks such as cooking, cleaning, washing, and polishing, they also dressed, undressed, and bathed the injured patients. As most of the young women involved hailed from well-to-do families, this was a huge step in their emancipation. Most would never before have been alone and unchaperoned with an unrelated member of the opposite sex.

The following is an extract from a message by Katharine Furse, Commandant-In-Chief, British Red Cross Society Women's Voluntary Aid Detachments, to VADs proceeding on active service;

You are being sent to work for the Red Cross. You have to perform a task which will need your courage, your energy, your patience, your humility, your determination to overcome all difficulties. Remember that the honour of the VAD organisation depends on your individual conduct. It will be your duty not only to set an example of discipline and perfect steadiness of character, but also to maintain the most courteous relations with those whom you are helping in this great struggle.

Be invariably courteous, unselfish and kind. Remember whatever duty you undertake, you must carry it out faithfully, loyally, and to the best of your ability.

Rules and regulations are necessary in whatever formation you join. Comply with them without grumble or criticism and try to believe that there is reason at the back of them, though at the time you may not understand the necessity.

Sacrifices may be asked of you. Give generously and wholeheartedly, grudging nothing, but remembering that you are giving because your Country needs your help. If you see others in better circumstances than yourself, be patient and think of the men who are fighting amid discomfort and who are often in great pain.

Those of you who are paid can give to the Red Cross Society, which is your Mother and which needs much more money to carry on its great work, to their Mother Society and thus to the Sick and Wounded.

Let our mottos be "Willing to do anything" and "The People give gladly". If we live up to these, the VAD members will come out of this world war triumphant.

Do your duty loyally
Fear God
Honour the King
And only the Master shall praise us, and only the Master shall blame.
And no one shall work for money, and no one shall work for fame.
But each for the joy of working, and each in his separate star,
Shall draw the thing as he sees it for the God of things as they are.

A PRAYER BY RACHEL CROWDY.

"Lord, who once bore your own Cross shoulder high to save mankind, help us to bear our Red Cross Banner high, with clean hands unafraid.

To those who tend the wounded and sick give health and courage that they of their store may give to those who lie awake in pain with strength and courage gone.

Teach us no task can be too great, no work too small, for those who die or suffer pain for us and their Country. Give unto those who rule a gentle justice and a wisely guiding hand, remembering "Blessed are the Merciful". And when peace comes, grant neither deed nor word of ours has thrown a shadow on the Cross, nor stained the flag of England".

(Note: The line 'Give unto those who rule a gentle justice and a wisely guiding hand' seems totally inappropriate when one considers the vast number of shell-shocked soldiers wrongly executed for cowardice).

Nurse Goodban appears to have commenced collecting for her book, which contains entries from more than one hundred of her patients, whilst at the Barnstaple VA Hospital in 1915 and continued until she finally left the Red Cross on January 31st 1919. It is possible that the autograph book may originally have been a gift to her from some of her grateful patients.

Herewith are excerpts from the book which are testament to the high regard in which she was held by those who benefited from her care and attention. Not all of her patients were gallant warriors wounded in action; some were ignominiously shipped home suffering from dysentery, trench fever, or trench foot but it is evident from the entries in her book that all her patients received the same level of devotion. The various entries on the pages display not only the gratitude felt for Nurse Goodban but also the mood of the British Tommy at the time. Despite the indescribable horrors that many had witnessed an unmistakeable air of humour and optimism prevails throughout the book. However, there is evidence that not every patient was without heartache; there are two poems which were obviously inspired by broken romances (See page 34).

CHAPTER ONE

BARNSTAPLE MILLER INSTITUTE/RED CROSS HOSPITAL

At various times in 1915, 1916, 1917, and 1918 Nurse Goodban worked in Barnstaple, North Devon. It is unclear from the records whether or not the Miller Institute and the Red Cross hospital were one and the same place. The following are entries made in her notebook during these times.

As all the entries were hand-written, some by severely maimed servicemen, not every word written could be understood. Where the signature could not be accurately ascertained an educated guess has been made of the surname. Such names are indicated with an asterisk throughout the book. Similarly, where the initial(s) are/is also in doubt, an asterisk has been placed by the doubtful one. Also, almost one hundred years ago, the standard of education varied enormously from man to man. To retain authenticity, wherever possible the words have been produced as they were written. Occasionally some minor spelling and punctuation mistakes have been rectified.

LEAVE

Now the day is over,
Leave is drawing nigh
Shadows of a dust up
Steal across the sky

No more weekly coalings
No more night defence
All the quids we have now
Are dwindling into pence.

Staying onboard so long now
Has made us rather glum
But that will soon get worked off
When with a "long haired chum"

But duty's coming nearer
For leave is getting short,
And soon we'll have a medal
For battles someone's fought.

Then a chap may ask you
What's that honour for?
"Wearing slacks in wartime"
Ought to stop his jaw.

Silence may be golden
And swearing indiscrete
Still they don't draft angels
To the British Fleet.

Though they don't draft angels
To the British Fleet
From Admiral to Snotty
They're all – well, simply sweet.

With kindest regards and best wishes to Nurse Goodban

Corporal R M Burn

This man describes himself as a corporal, which is not a naval rank, and yet he writes about the British Fleet and being 'on board'. Maybe he was a marine?

I was wounded in france a place call Hooge wounded in the right fore arm on the 6 of july 1915 i have been out there since last May 1914 and wounded once i was sent out of the trenches down to the dressing station I was there for one night and then sent to Trypots from there sent to Exeter wear i resied (*possibly "received" – author*) many thanks from the nurses and the Sister and then sent to the Red Cross Hospital Barnstaple were i resied every bit of kindness from the nurses.

Private G E Samwell.
1st Royal Foresters

Wounded at the Dardanelles. A small word – with a large Bearing "Thanks"
12th October 1915

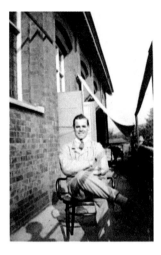

Private Victor Ellwood
Duke of Wellingtons

Invalided home from the Dardanelles with Dysentery and Neuralgia was transferred from Plymouth to Barnstaple Institute where I am almost got well again. Best wishes to all the nurses there and good luck to all.

Private H Haylett
1/5 Norfolks

Rendered "Hors-de-combat" at Dardanelles 21st August 1915.

Trooper A F Chapman
Middlesex Hussars

Sent home with Dysentery from Dardanelles 17th September 1915.

Private R Armstrong
1st Royal Inniskillen Fusiliers

With many thanks for the kind treatment received at Red Cross Hospital Barnstaple.

11th October 1915
Pte Brumbill
1/1st Herefords Regt

Greater love hath no man than this, that a man lay down his own life for his friends.
Wounded at Dardanelles on 28th June 1915

From Yours Aye Jock
Rifleman Thomas Ferguson 2202

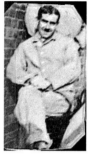

(Scottish Rifles) Cameronians.

Wounded at Sulva Bay, Dardanelles August 13th 1915.

Pte Gordon A. Browne
1/5 Norfolk Regt

The Dardanelles offensive, better known as the Gallipoli Campaign, lasted from February 1915 until January 1916 and can only truthfully be regarded as an unmitigated disaster. Military and naval commanders were totally opposed to the action but politicians, including Winston Churchill, in response to a request from Grand Duke Nicholas the commander of the Russian armies, ordered the offensive to go ahead.

The intention was to land a combined force of British, French, and Commonwealth soldiers to attack and defeat the Turkish Army and then march into Constantinople. In so doing they would relieve pressure on the Russians on the Caucasus front. The action commenced with a naval bombardment of the Turkish positions. However, owing to a totally unexpected show of resistance, the action resulted in the loss of three ships and three other craft damaged. Subsequent land battles resulted in 213,980 Commonwealth casualties before the campaign was abandoned. The renowned war poet Rupert Brooke was a casualty of the Gallipoli Campaign having died of blood poisoning from a mosquito bite en route to the front. It seems rather an inglorious death for a man who had written so much of war and its aftermath.

There was a man who could not speak
Of course this was no joke
He went into the joiners shop
Picked up a Chisel and Spoke.

With best wishes
Private A Maybin
7th Batt East Surrey
Lest We Forget

Just a few lines_____

_____

_____

From a shy young man.
Wounded 25th Sept 1915
Wounded 1st July 1916

With best wishes to Nurse Goodban

Pte L. Cook 948
2nd Queens R.W.S.

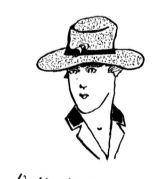

With best wishes from Ex Private R J Gregory.
23rd July 1917.

*(It appears that this man is anxious to point out that he already considers
himself demobbed! He also has a second entry in the book. See page 40)*

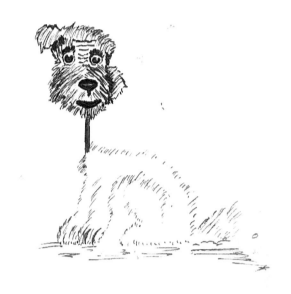

My Little Wet Home in the Trench

My little wet home in the trench
That's the place where we fright with the French
The Germans they know, so you have to keep low,
In my little wet home in the trench.
There is no-one to visit you there,
For the place is so muddy and bare,
But I've got one good friend I can trust to the end
In my little dug-out in the trench.

My rifle's the only defence,
If that should refuse, then perhaps I might lose
My little dug-out in the trench.
But still I should never say die
For my comrades will always stand by,
The shots they come swift
But still none of us shift
From our little dug-out in the trench.

In my little dug-out in the trench
When I'm in it it makes me feel dense,
But still I don't mind when I sit down to eat
In my little dug-out in the trench.
When the guns are booming around
And the shells are ploughing the ground
With shells dropping near I shall never fear
In my little dug-out in the trench.

A sniper sat up in a tree
I saw he was sniping at me
I fired a shot and it was a cold pot
From my little dug-out in the trench.
As the Huns they come dashing along,
The lads strike up with a song
And the gunners they know that the lads will not go
From their little dug-outs in the trench.

Old England a victory will win,
You'll see when the movement begin,
The gunners will go with their heads hanging low
From their little dug-outs in the trench.
If only this war was to cease
And the sound of that little word peace
With fast beating heart I would willingly part
With my little wet home in the trench.

Wounded at Poizieres (Albert) by shrapnel in the shoulder and thigh 1st July 1916 (Big Push)

With my sincere wishes for a greater success in your glorious work you are now doing, and many, many thanks for your kindness to me whilst in hospital.

> "When the wind blows then the mill goes
> May it grind you golden grain.
> May your lifetime run in the light of the sun
> And all your days be gain"

> Believe me, yours sincerely

> Private F H Reid
> 2nd Middlesex Regt
> (Die Hards!)

Nurse Goodban with patients at Barnstaple, North Devon.

Standing; Pte Kermode, Cpl R M Burn, Nurse Passmore, Frances Goodban, Melhuish

Sitting: Foster, Gunner Brewster, Manning, plus Togo the dog.

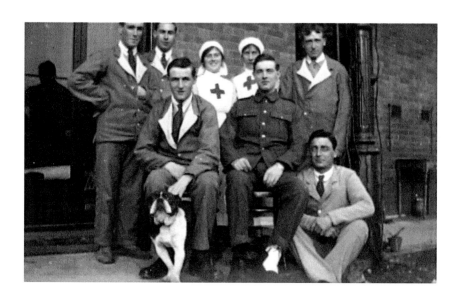

Nurse Goodban with patients at Barnstaple, North Devon.

Standing: Pte A Walsh, Sgt Thomas, Frances Goodban, Trooper H Venables, Pte Joe Morley
Sitting: Pte Clark, unknown.

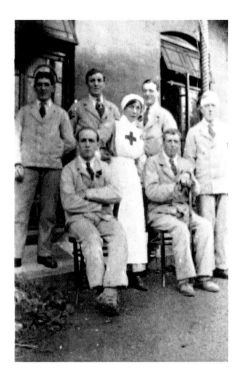

Nurse Goodban with patients at Barnstaple, North Devon.

Standing: Pte A Walsh, Sgt Thomas, Driver McConaghy, Trooper H Venables, Pte Joe Morley
Sitting; Pte Clarke, Unknown

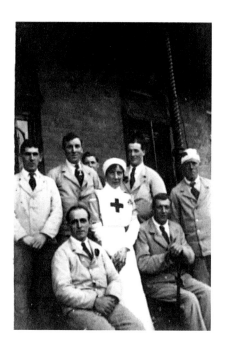

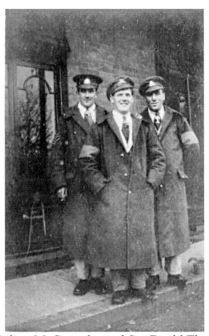

CQMS J Walker, Driver McConaghy and Sgt David Thomas at Barnstaple.

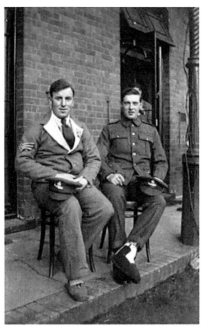

Sergeant Thomas and Gunner Brewster at Barnstaple

Patients at Barnstaple, North Devon.

Back row; Cpl R M Burn, Foster, Melhuish
Middle row: Sgt David Anthony Thomas, Manning
Front row: Gunner Brewster, CQMS Walker, Pte G N Kermode

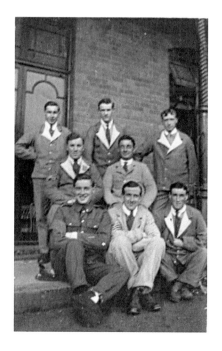

Message on drawing.

Miss Gladizeck.

With Best Wishes to Nurse Goodban.
C.Q.M.Sgt J. Walker
11th Bttn East Lancs Regt.

England, dear England, the land of my birth,
I'm proud of thy freedom, thy beauty, and worth.
Where ever I may wander, by land or sea,
Oxford, dear Oxford, my heart is with thee.

Gassed in the Big Push 1916

Every sincere wish from
Rifleman S E Haynes*
The Rifle Brigade

Although with smiles they entered the field
Determined that they would not yield
But alas their fate was sealed (and today)
But next time a better show
They may make it for all we know
If their men will show more go
Let us pray.

Lance Corporal H Stanley
94th Field Company R.E.

The Limit
"Annexation"
Is vexation.
"Reparation", is as bad,
"Indemnity"
Doth puzzle me -
And "Peace Talk" drives me mad.

Best wishes to Nurse Goodban

Sergeant D A Thomas
R H A

So let us pray that comes it may
As come it will for a' that,
That sense and worth o'er all the earth
May bear the gree and a'that,
It's coming yet for a'that
That man to man the world o'er
Shall brothers be for a' that.

Wha'd thought it – Wha's like us!

L/ Corporal John Steel
Royal Scots Fusiliers
Beith, Ayrshire, Scotland

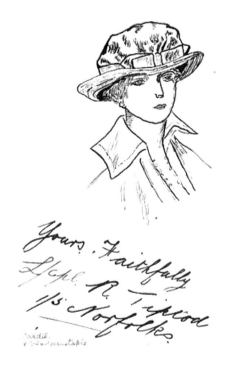

Message reads;

Yours faithfully
L/Cpl. Tiptod
1/5 Norfolks

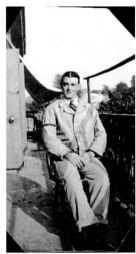

Lance Corporal Tiptod

A nice little Blighty
Makes a nice little Rest
In a nice little Hospital
Down in the West

> Private J Bentley
> 7 North Derbys

If the rich would part with money
Like poor mothers do with sons
This war would soon be over
Instead blood freely runs.
Best wishes

> Lance Corporal P J Quirke*
> 1st Royal Dublin Fusiliers

Wounded in the battle for Loos 24th September 1915 but thanks to the Sisters and Nurses of the Red Cross Hospital Barnstaple I am got quite fit again. Wishing them all the very best of luck. 16th November 1915

> Sergeant E F Nash
> 1st Gloucestershire Regiment

Stick it the Welsh! Shrapnel wound of face September 25th 1915 in France. Many thanks to the Sisters and Nurses of No 4 ward Barnstaple. November 16th 1915

> Wishing them good luck
> Private G Thomas
> 9 Welsh Regiment

Wounded at Vermelles in the right knee with shrapnel on the eighth of October 1915. Many thanks to the Sisters and Nurses of No 4 Ward for their kind attention. 16th November 1915

> Lance Corporal T Riess
> 6th R W Kent Regiment

Wounded at the Great Advance at "Loos" bullet through right arm. Thanks to the Sisters and Nurses for their kind treatment. 6th November 1915

> Corporal J. Hamilton
> 1st Batt Black Watch

Wounded in France by shrapnel on the 25th September 1915 at the battle of Loos, was in hospital in France for three weeks then came to Barnstaple. Many thanks to the Sisters and Nurses of this hospital. 16th November 1915

Lance Corporal J Kilgour
9th Black Watch

Landed in France 25th November 1914. Got wounded through the right arm at Givenchy on the 10th October 1915. It is better now thanks to the Sisters, nurses of the Red Cross Hospital Barnstaple. November 16th 1915

Corporal F* Solly
2nd Borderers

Wounded in a charge for a position at the base of the slagheaps, a name given to several large hills of small coal lying between Vermelles and Hulloch. The wounds received were, Shrapnel in the left shoulder, and a dum-dum bullet in the right leg. I am almost well now, thanks to the clever sister of ward no. 4 of Barnstaple Hospital and the kind attention of Nurse Goodban, to whom I am indebted. 16th November 1915

Private H Butler
3rd Dragoon Guards
Attched to 2nd Batt The Buffs.

Most, if not all, of the men listed on the previous fifteen pages were injured in the "Big Push" or "Great Advance" that took place in the autumn of 1915. It became known as The Battle of Loos and for many of Kitchener's Army – the wartime recruits – it was their first experience of major warfare. After two and a half weeks of bitter fighting, 20,000 British soldiers lay dead. Many were the sons of illustrious figures such as politicians and aristocrats who had joined up midst the fervour of patriotism; others were famous in their own right. The battle was a failure insomuch as it did not put an end to trench warfare as had been its intended aim.

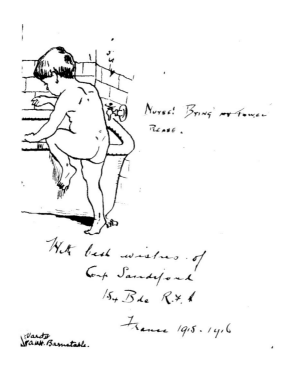

Message reads;

With best wishes of
Corp Sandiford
154 Bde R. F. R.
France 1915 – 1916

Mountains of beef
Rivers of beer
Nice little wife
And a £1000 a year.   Wounded on 1st June 1916

19th September 1916
Private E Millard
9th East Surreys

Wounded at Hebutune June 20th 1916.
26th Sept 1916

George Wiseman
MT ASC

A Noisy Noise

When bombs are hurtling everywhere
And bursting in wild wrath,
When hissing shrieks invade the air
And cannon, belching forth
Their deadly missiles everywhere
Boom West, South, East, and North.
When yells rise from a thousand boys
Who've won a trench
– Well, that's a noise!

Wounded at Hebuterne 16th June 1916

Private J Forbes*
1st Kensington Battalion

"In whatever has been made by the Deity externally delighted to the human sense of beauty, there is some type of God's laws"   Ruskin

Wounded at Fricourt July 1st 1916

Cpl F Hirst
10th Batt. Yorks and Lancs Regt

When seas and hills divide us
And you no more I see
Remember it was Benson
That wrote these lines for thee

Wounded July 11th 1916

Pte J. J Benson
2nd Bedford Regt

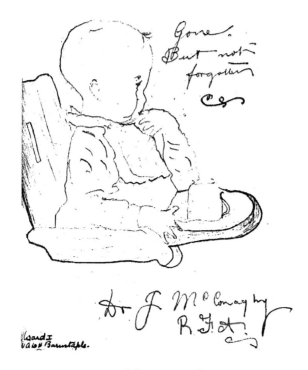

Message reads;
Gone but not forgotten

Driver J. McConaghy
R.F.A.

When the golden sun is setting,
And your mind from care is free
When of others you are thinking
Will you sometimes think of me?

26th August 1916

Rifleman T Dudley
The Rifle Brigade

Invalided home with Trench Fever and sent to Barnstaple Red Cross Hospital where I received every kindness and attention from the nurses. With many thanks.
27th August 1916

Rifleman W Ashley
The Rifle Brigade

Louis J Wells, his mark "X"   Wounded Gommecourt July 1st 1916

This entry is intriguing. Why just an "X" as a signature? Was the man illiterate or could he not write because of the extent of his injuries? Also why no rank or regiment?

Conquer we shall, but we must first contend
T'is not the fight that crowns us, but the end!
Wounded at Gommecourt 1st July 1916 (Somme Push)

With best wishes and thanks. Sincerely yours

Vincent E Robbins
1st Queen Victoria's Rifles

When pain and anguish wring the brow
A ministering angel thou.
29th August 1916

Wounded at Gommecourt 1st July 1916

Rifleman F C Phillips
1st Queen's Westminster Rifles

It's rather funny
It makes me laugh
When I think what to put
For my autograph.   20th September 1916

T R Kightley
Royal Field Artillery

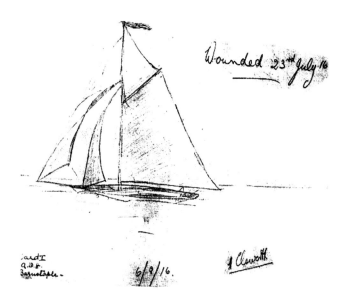

Message reads:
Wounded 23rd July 1916

H.* Elsworth

6th Sept 1916

"It is not the length of existence that counts but what is achieved during that existence"

The machine gun is an invention of the devil. (How well the Germans know it)
Wounded at Neuve Chapelle 10th August 1916
20th September 1916

Private S C Sadler
Machine Gun Corps
"Cymru Am Byth"

Fall from a chimney top
Fall from above
Fall from a house top
But don't fall in love.
Wounded 18th August 1915 and 1st July 1916

27th August 1916
L/Cpl G Watton
1/5thNorth Staffs Regt

Here's to the train that runs on time
And never, never sights danger.
Here's to the girl that sticks to one chap
And never runs off with a stranger.

25th September 1916

With Best Wishes to Nurse Goodban

Private G Lister*
16th West Yorks

It is apparent from the preceding two entries that the wounds suffered by the patients were not only to their bodies. They both appear to have suffered heartache in their recent pasts. Being a war hero was obviously not a guarantee of having a faithful lover. Indeed, the very act of being a hero could have caused the break-up in their relationships. Maybe their injuries or disfigurement was too much for their partner to bear.

*Many of the men on the previous few pages were injured on the Somme, a river in Picardy, North West France. The Battle of the Somme lasted from 1st July 1916 until 18th November 1916 at the end of which the British had suffered 420,000 casualties (60,000 on the first day!). The French army sustained 200,000 casualties and the Germans half a million. **It is officially one of the bloodiest battles ever recorded in history.***

The aim of the advance against the well dug-in German forces, who had occupied a lot of France since August 1914, was to drag enemy re-enforcements from the battle at Verdun where the French were being hard pressed by the Germans. The plan, as so many early allied plans did, failed miserably.

The British Tommies, volunteers to a man and many seeing action for the first time, were sent into battle weighed down with a plethora of equipment. Besides their weapons each man carried two gas masks, wire cutters, a shovel, 220 rounds of ammunition, a ground sheet, a haversack, field dressings, and two sand bags. A total load of seventy pounds!

They were ordered to proceed towards the enemy positions line abreast; sitting, or more likely waddling ducks for the German machine gunners. Thousands were mown down in the first five minutes. Their bodies provided the only cover for the troops bringing up the rear. Even the Germans were so appalled by the carnage that on the following two mornings they held an impromptu four hour cease fire to allow stretcher parties to collect the injured. It eventually took three days to collect them all. By November the French and British forces had advanced seven miles; a loss of 88,000 men for every mile.

*At the outset of the battle the British military commanders held a full regiment of cavalry in reserve ready to charge into the hole in the enemy lines. Fortunately, the hole never materialised as one could only imagine the fate of both horses and riders galloping into the barbed wire, trenches, shell holes, and the withering fire from the German machine guns. It is no surprise at all that the German military chiefs described the British army of the time as **"lions led by donkeys"**.*

At this time of the war the British Army was mostly a volunteer force with many battalions made up from men of specific local areas. The loss of countless thousands of young men from such communities had a profound social impact which was to be felt for decades after hostilities ended. One place in particular that was badly affected was the Dominion of Newfoundland. A huge number of Newfoundland volunteers were lost on the first day of the battle.

The battle is also remembered in the annuals of war as the first time that tanks were actually used in warfare.

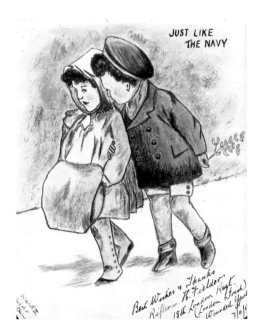

Message reads;
Best Wishes and Thanks

Rifleman H. Fielder
18th London Regt
(London Irish)

Wounded Ypres 7th April 1917

He Did The Deed
With face impurled (sic), lips compressed
He seems just like a man possessed
Uncanny Mutt'rings from him came
His eyes were like two stars of flame.
Determination wild and grim
Was written large all over him
"Ye Gods!" he shouted with a sigh,
"I'll do it – yes – I will – or die!"
Within his hand a knife he bore
He tried its blunted edge once more,
And did it. Yes, it wanted pluck
To carve that antiquated duck!   Wounded 7th June 1917 at Messines.

Thanking Nurse Goodban for her kindness to me during my stay in Ward 3 VA
Hospital, Barnstaple also wishing her a bright and happy future.

Lance Corporal M Johnson
2nd Bttln, Royal Irish Regiment

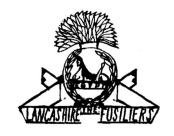

Wounded. Messeins
June 7th 1917.
Pte. W. Ardern.

Ward III
V.A.D.H. Barnstaple

Wounded Messines, 7th June 1917

Pte W Ardern
Lancashire Fusiliers

May luck be yours. Many thanks to Nurse Goodban for her kindness to me at the VA Hospital.
7th July 1917

Private B Elsworth 44019
9th Kings Own Yorkshire Light Infantry

Thanking Nurse Goodban for the kindness and attention to me whilst at VA Hospital, Barnstaple.

10th July 1917

Lance Corporal GW Nobbs 4008
1st Queen Victoria Rifles
9th London Regimen

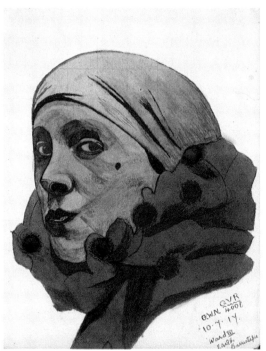

Inscription reads:
G.W.N.   Q.V.R.   4008

10/7/1917

Give me a friend who varies not or else no friend at all,
Who'll love me in my humble cot as in my marble hall.
Who'll chide me when I do amiss
Who'll praise me when praise is due,
Who'll help me in my sightlessness
And be forever true.

23rd July 1917
Ex Private R J Gregory
Late 8th Devons

I found this poem particularly poignant. Does his reference to "sightlessness" refer to loss of an eye, or both? The fact that he deliberately points out that he considers himself already discharged from the army is also unusual. Men were generally discharged after leaving hospital not whilst still a patient.

I'll note you in my memory ear (?) - Tennyson.

Thanking Nurse Goodban for kind attention and treatment while at VA Hospital, Barnstaple.
(28th August 1917)

Corporal A C Bennett
1/5th Gloucesters

Little puffs of powder;
Little drops of paint;
Makes the Lady's face;
What it really ain't;

Nurse Goodban, I shall never forget your kindness and careful attention to me during the time which I have spent in Barnstaple VA Hospital. I can assure you I appreciate your kindness to me and cannot thank you sufficiently.
With best wishes and thanks to Nurse Goodban

Wounded at Ypres Sept 28th 1917

Gunner A Brewster
D/5 Battery RFA

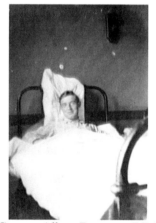

Gunner Albert Brewster RFA

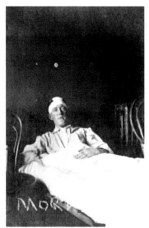

Private Joe Morley at Barnstaple Red Cross Hospital

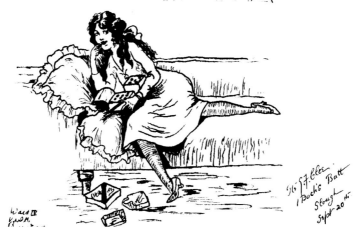

Message reads: Chocolates are easy to pack.

Pte G.F.Clee
1 Bucks Battalion
Slough
Sept 20th (1916?)

Nurse Goodban, I shall always remember no matter where ere I may be for her kindness, it is unlimited. Her equals are hard to find. God grant; She may be rewarded for all she is doing today.
With best wishes and thanks,
23rd October 1917

Trooper H Venables
6th Inniskillen Dragoons

It's a good thing to smile
When life flows along like a song,
But the man worth while
Is the man who will smile
When everything goes dead wrong.
For the world is full of sorrow
And sorrow comes along with years
But the smile that is worth all the praise in the world
Is the smile that comes through tears.

With kindest regards and best wishes to Nurse Goodban. 5th December 1917
Private G N Kermode

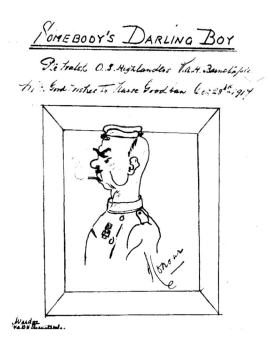

Message reads;
SOMEBODY'S DARLING BOY

Private Walsh   A. S. Highlanders   V.A.H. Barnstaple
With Good Wishes to Nurse Goodban   October 28th 1917
Best wishes from unreadable E---------, H   Private 17491

From his Army number it should be simple to trace this patient.

CHAPTER TWO

NETLEY RED CROSS HOSPITAL near Southampton

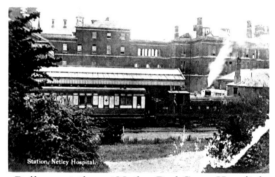
Railway station at Netley Red Cross Hospital

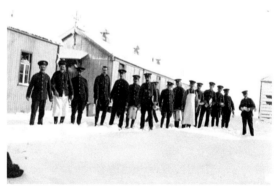
"Tea up" at Netley Red Cross Hospital

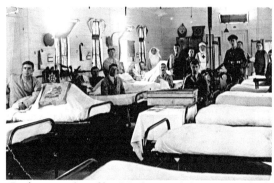
Patients and staff at Netley Red Cross Hospital

From left to right: Pte H. Gee, Orderly Lauder, Pte Peter Aitkin, Cpl T G Hughes, Sister Ripper, Willard, Gunner G. Becker, Pte R. Bainbridge, Pte A H Binns, Gunner Hutton, Aitkinson, Unknown Lieutenant, Orderly, Richmond, Unknown.

Seriously wounded servicemen would have been shipped to Southampton docks from the battle zones of France, Belgium, the Dardanelles, and even Mesopotamia. Netley Red Cross hospital would therefore have had a crucial role in initially treating these men who were then often sent on to other hospitals for further treatment and convalescence.

I ain't nobody's Sweetheart yet!

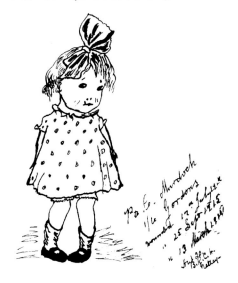

Message reads;

Wounded 17th July 1915
Wounded 25th September 1915
Wounded 13th March 1916

Pte E Murdoch
1/4 * Gordons

It seems it was a case of third time lucky for this Scots soldier!

Still swinging the lead.
Wounded in France January 13th 1916.

Pte D. Shayler*
11th Royal Fusiliers

With Good Wishes to Sisters and Nurses at Netley Hospital.
Wounded April 15th 1915 Ypres
Gassed July 4th 1916
Sent home sick Feb 2nd 1917

Cpl S J Gallagher
9 Battalion Tyneside Scottish

With many thanks for the kindness received at the Red Cross Hospital Netley.

E. Travers
6th Dragoons

The last mentioned soldiers were just a sample of the many thousands that were casualties of the war in Flanders. The red poppy that is sold before Remembrance Day in the UK is based on the abundance of poppies that grow wild to this day in the fields of Northern France and the Belgian border. The area is famous for its breweries and the poppies can often be seen flourishing amongst the many hop vines.

There were three major battles fought in this area, namely Ypres, known to the Tommies as 'Wipers', (October/November1914), Passchendaele (July – November 1917), and Lys (April 1918). There was in reality almost a continuous fight for Ypres with at least four different battles on record but the major one was early in the war in 1914.

Ypres was important to both sides as it was the gateway to the Channel ports, especially Dunkirk and Calais which were essential to keep supply lines up and running. The Allies eventually won a decisive victory but not without substantial losses. Of the original 160,000 soldiers of the British Expeditionary Force who fought more than half were killed, injured, or taken prisoner. However, what was devastating was the fact that the British Army witnessed the destruction of its highly trained and experienced regular army. Conversely, the German army had been made up of reserves most of which were totally inexperienced. The German losses totalled 150,000 and the battle was known as **Kindermord bei Ypern** – the Battle of the Innocents- thereafter.

The Battle of Passchendaele was one of the major battles of this campaign. Passchendaele has become synonymous with the misery of relentless struggle for virtually no gain. Fighting took place quite often in waist deep mud. Men and horses actually drowned in the stuff. To further exacerbate matters the summer of 1917 was unusually wet and cold.

It was the Canadian Corps who eventually captured the town from the Germans by which time the Allies had lost 140,000 men; a ratio of one dead man for every two inches (five centimetres) of ground gained. Five months later at the Battle of Lys the Germans regained the same ground without much resistance.

The debate still rages over whether or not the price paid for victory was worth it. At the time David Lloyd George, the then Prime Minister, stated that it was a senseless waste of life and an example of poor generalship. Conversely, it is argued that by inflicting heavy losses on the Germans, relieving pressure on the French Forces, and developing defensive tactics, the Allies were better equipped to later win the war.

The Battle of Lys was nothing compared to the previous two Flanders Battles and remarkable only for the fact that the Portuguese 2nd Division of 20,000 men lost 300 officers and 7,000 men killed, wounded, or taken prisoner.

Wounded in France July 1st 1916. Went to 7 Canadian General Hospital for a month then came to British Red X Hospital. Many thanks to the Doctors and Sisters and Nurses for their kind attention to me at Netley British Red Cross Hospital.

7th December 1916
Pte J T Dudley
6th Notts

Here's luck to the sailor on board of ship
Here's luck to the soldier on sentry
Here's luck to the woman that is doing their bit
For the sake of their king and country
Wounded 1st July 1916 at Warnatz (?) France

11th November 1916

Pte T.Preddy
9th Devons

Wounded 26th Feb 1916 in Somme Push.

L/Cpl E A Kaminski
8 Canadian Lt Inf Batt

Wounded 26th September 1916 at Somme Push.

P W Pietrowski
15 Canadian Lt Inf

Wounded 3rd July 1916

Pte B Andrews
9th Essex Regt

Wounded at Somme (Trones Wood) July 14th 1916. Gunshot wound left leg. Thanks to the splendid nursing in the B. Red X Hospital, Netley, I am speedily recovering.

With good wishes to Nurse Goodban.

L/Cpl H. House
12th Middlesex Regt
(Die Hards)

The rose is red,
The violets blue,
Honeys sweet,
And so are you.

With best wishes to Nurse Goodban.

Wounded at Trones Wood on the Somme July 25th 1916.
10th November 1916

Pte W Bullock
Machine Gun Corps

Military Manoeuvres – and Otherwise.

"Bang!" went the rifles at the manoeuvres.
"Ooooh" screamed a pretty girl.
A nice, decorous, surprised little scream.
She slipped backwards into the arms of a young man.
"Oh" she said, blushing, "I was frightened by the rifles. I beg your pardon"
"Not at all" said the young man, "Let's go over and watch the artillery". And
they did.

Wounded in the big push on the Somme 26th September 1916 just south of
Thiepval. Gunshot wounds left thigh and arms. Thanks to the doctors and good
nursing am fast recovering.

Pte R C Sellers
10th Canadian Infantry

A Yorkshire man's advice to his son.

Hear all, see all, and say nowt,
Ate all, drink all, and pay nowt,
Never thee do owt for nowt,
If ever tha does owt for nowt,
Do it for thee sen.

With best wishes and thanks to Nurse Goodban for her kindness to me.
Invalided from the Somme October 10th 1916.

Gnr A Hutton*
66th S Btty RGA

If wisdom's ways you'd wisely seek
Five things observe with care,
Of whom you speak, to whom you speak,
And how, and when, and where.
Wounded at Delville Wood October 28th 1916

Pte R. Bainbridge
22nd Durham Lt Infantry

Yet again we have many soldiers who were wounded on the Somme (see page 36). It is no wonder this battle is considered one of the bloodiest in history.

At various times all the hospitals that Nurse Goodban worked in had patients who were being treated for injuries sustained in the Somme campaign.

When this you see
Just think of me
When I've left England's shore
For when I've gone
To fight the hun
I'll think of you the more.

With best wishes. Invalided from Macedonia with trench feet 23rd October 1916.

5830 Pte H Gee
13th Manchester Regt

Poor Tommy

Give him strong drink until he winks and sinking in despair,
And liquor good to fire his blood and sooth his griefs and cares,
Let him booze in deep carouse
With bumpers flowing o'er
Till he forgets his love and shells and thinks of them no more.

Delighted with Nurse Goodban's attention. Gallipoli and Mesopotamia.
11th November 1916

Pte N Durkin
Loyal North Lancs

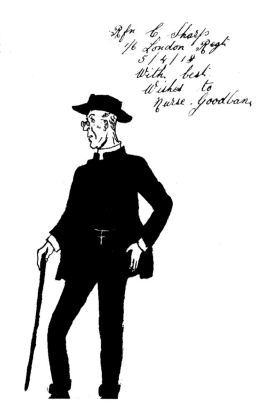

Message reads;

Rifleman C. Sharp
1/6 London Regiment
5th April 1918

With best wishes to Nurse Goodban

Ah! How easily things go wrong –
A kiss too much, a sigh too long.
Then comes the mist and the weeping rain
And the world is never the same again.
Wounded in Mesopotamia.

With all good wishes to Sisters and Nurses.

15919 Pte F Taylor
2nd Dorsets
6 Poona Division

The two previous soldiers were wounded in the campaign against the Turks in Mesopotamia, which is now in modern day Iraq. The 6th Poona Division, led by Major General Townshend, consisted of British and Indian Army soldiers, some13,000 men in total.

The unit landed at Basra with the aim of marching north to capture Baghdad. At the first meeting with the Turkish Army at Ctesiphon the Allies were successful but suffered heavy casualties; Privates Durkin and Taylor were probably just two of them. The much depleted 6th Poona Division retreated to Kut-a-Amara, a town sited on a loop of the River Tigris, in December 1915. However, this proved to be a mistake of momentous proportions as the only way back out of the town was quickly blocked and surrounded by over 10,000 Turkish troops. Townshend and his men could do nothing but sit tight and await a relief force and supplies. However, none were forthcoming.

Two relief columns were sent out, the first of which was led by Sir Fenton Aylmer. The column was repeatedly repulsed by the Turks with heavy losses sustained at Sheikh Sa'ad, Wadi, Hanna, and Dujaila. A second column led by General Gorringe was also unable to fight its way through the enemy lines. An attempt to re-supply by way of the river was thwarted by a Turkish blockade and the paddle steamer Junlar was captured. During the abortive relief attempts the British suffered a further 23,000 casualties.

In desperation Townshend was authorised to offer a million pounds plus a guarantee that none of his men would fight again against the Turks. Khalil Pasha, the Military Governor of Baghdad, was agreeable to the offer but was overruled by the Minister of War Enver Pasha who demanded an unconditional surrender.

After a siege of 143 days, during which time the British troops were reduced to killing and eating their own horses, the garrison laid down their arms and surrendered. Many of the Indian Army soldiers, being Hindus, had refused to eat horse meat and had consequently died of starvation. A large percentage of the soldiers taken prisoner, both British and Indian, also died after being brutally treated by their captives.

The quality of mercy is not strained
It droppeth as the gentle rain from Heaven
Upon the place beneath.
It is twice blessed,
It blesseth him that giveth and him that taketh.

In grateful remembrance of the many kindnesses received.
December 1916

Sapper C J Lane
Royal Engineers "Signals"

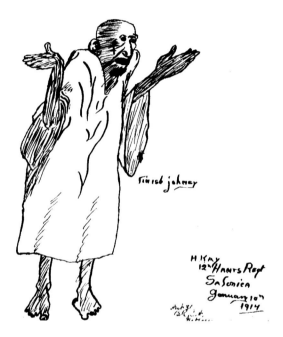

The message reads;

FINISH JOHNEY

H. Kay
12th Hampshire Regiment
Salonica
January 10th 1917

Just a few words to express my gratitude for the great care and kindness shown
to me by Nurse Goodban while I was in Ward 31 BRC Hospital, Netley.

Wounded at Levante on the 23rd January 1917.

Rfn A O Harris – James
1st Queen's Westminster Rifles.

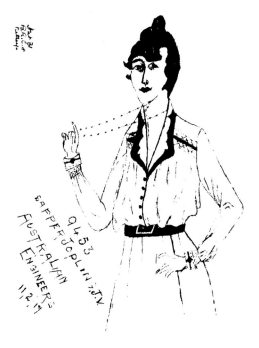

Message reads;

Sapper Jopling J.V. 9453
Australian Engineers   11th February 1917

Many thanks to Nurse Goodban for her kindness shown to me while at the Red Cross Hospital Netley.
16th February 1917

Cpl T M* Hughes
Coldstream Guards

With many thanks to Nurse Goodban for the care and kindness shown to me while in Hut 31, British Red Cross Hospital Netley.
Pte Bert A Foot
LMG

7th London Regt
"Shiny Seventh"

April 1917

T'is the one who's full of sunshine, and genuinely tries,
Who will clear the clouds of trouble from her own and other's skies.
Deeds of honest loving-kindness give a fallen fellow heart,
And upon his uphill journey help him play a manly part.

To Nurse Goodban for her great kindness during my stay.

20th February 1917

G. Becker
121st Siege Battery
RGA

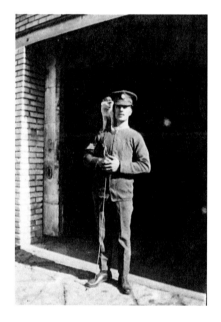

Message reads;

"Guess which is ME"

Sergeant Pittaway M.G.
A.S.C.S.

1st July

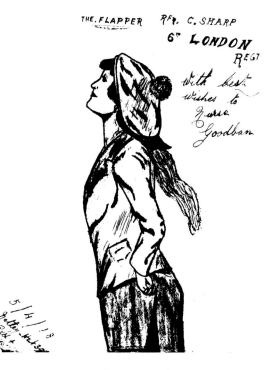

Message reads:
THE FLAPPER

Rifleman C. Sharpe
6th London regiment

With best wishes to Nurse Goodban. 5th April 1918

Hope on, hope ever, joy cometh in the morning,
It is ever the darkest before dawn.
Life is not a goblet to be drained but rather a measure to be filled.
If you cannot realise yours ideas, idealise your reals.

With kind thoughts and best wishes to Nurse Goodban for services rendered.

Pte H Slack
124 Lab Company
16th Queens Regiment

Not every patient was an artist or poet, as demonstrated here:

Robinson "Scooted it". May 1st 1918

Bdr Walker C. "Rumbled" May 3rd 1918

Gunner Walker E. "Rumbled" May 3rd 1918

L/Cpl Nicholson J. "Hopped it" May 3rd 1918

Best wishes to Nurse Goodban.

32816 Driver Lund H.
64th Battery
RFA

The rank 'driver' here most probably does not apply to the driving of motor vehicles; it is more than likely that he drove horses. It has been estimated that 6 to 8 million horses were utilised by the various armies in the war. At the end of hostilities only some 62,000 were still alive.

The horses were used to transport food, ammunition, and troops and loads of 130 kilograms (around 20 stone) were normal. The animals also had to haul guns, often through thick mud. Mules were also used and both animals were extremely underfed most of the time.

At one time during the campaign the British Army were purchasing 15,000 horses a month just to replace ones killed in battle.

There have been several monuments erected around Europe to commemorate the extraordinary debt owed to these magnificent creatures.

"With my best wishes for the way I have been treated by Nurse Goodban. I will never forget the day that I arrived at the British Red Cross Hospital"

(Translated from French)   13th May 1918

416379 Pte H Gauthier
22nd French Canadian Battalion

This is just one of many non-British soldiers who were treated at Red Cross hospitals in the UK.

NETLEY

By Southampton water
Flanked by shady trees,
Stands Mercy's greatest daughter
The home of rest and ease.

For the maimed and broken
In Armageddon's fight,
Who with deeds unspoken
Have fought defending Right.

Where medicos and nurses
Each strive their best to heal
And the Public's open purses
On comforts put their seal.

Victoria, Welsh, and Netley Red Cross
You'll live in history,
You've proved you're gold – not dross
Their Blessed Trinity.

Through this world's commotion
You have stood the strain,
Not for gain or promotion
But Love's triumph over Pain.

Spr Rackham
Royal Engineers

18th May 1918

When War is at Hand
And danger's nigh,
God and the Soldier
Is all the cry.
When War is over
And all things righted
God is Forgotten
And the Soldier slighted.

F. Rock

(No rank or regiment mentioned but I feel sure the man was a soldier)

29th June 1918

I wish you Health, I wish you Wealth, I wish you Gold in Store,
I wish you Heaven when you die, What can I wish you more?

The Nurse
She hasn't a Sword and hasn't a gun,
But She's doing her duty Now fighting's begun.

(The sergeant's literary skills earned him two entries!)
29th June 1918

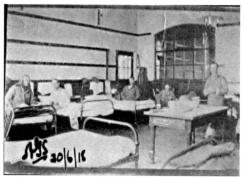

AJS is Sergeant Skinner. No further information

Sgt A J Skinner
1st Battalion
Rifle Brigade

Thanks to Nurse Goodban for her kindness, and gratefulness while with Ward 33.

30th June 1918

724 Pte A G Stafford
5 Australian Machine Gun Battalion AGF

Just a line to remember me
When I am gone far o'er the sea.

537 Pte P Aitkin
30th Battalion
8th Brigade
Australian Forces

The two previous entries were from just a couple of the many wounded Australian soldiers treated at Red Cross Hospitals.

Nothing was a trouble, even extra blanket, hot water bottle, or "buckshee" cup of tea.

My very best wishes for future happiness and sincere thanks for many kindnesses during my *camouflaged* state. Hoping other honours besides that of "sergeants" may soon wander your way.
Ps May the Spanish Flu and you never be friends.
2nd July 1918

Spr D. Borthwick
Royal Engineers Telegraphs

I can only assume by his camouflaged state that the soldier above was referring to the dressings which covered him; possibly his entire face.

His mention of "sergeants" seems to imply that Nurse Goodban was to be moved to a Senior NCO's ward. The British Army has always been rank conscious with distinct separation between junior ranks, senior ranks, and officers. This "promotion" is also borne out by the fact that some future entries are by men of the rank of sergeant.

The Spanish Flu mentioned by Sapper Borthwick had worked its way from the Far East, especially China and India, into Europe by the middle of 1918. It eventually arrived in Britain in September of that year. Millions of people died, especially troops weakened by years of fighting and poor nutrition. The US Federal Bureau of Health declared that more American troops died of the flu' than by enemy action.

When this you see just think of me
When I am far away
Across the sea
I'll think of thee
And will come back to you some day.

Taylor Frank

Again here no rank or regiment. Also not sure if name is Taylor Frank or Frank Taylor.

With many thanks for your kind attention. Best wishes for your future welfare.

Pte P J Truss   2073162
1st Infantry ASC

Words fail me in expression for the kindness and care shown during my stay here by the Sisters and Nurse Goodban. May happy thoughts be yours and happier days in store.

Pte A H Binns
LMG
1/6 West Yorks Regt

One of the boys.

H. Horsham
Hillside
Bosq Lane Guernsey

This man obviously could not wait to put his military past behind him! He has omitted any rank or regiment and even included his home address.

If one's luck receives a tumble
After aspirations high,
The disappointed must not grumble
Whether you or whether I.

6th November to 29th December 1917

Sgt Burridge L*
Irish Guards

Steady Cameroons steady,
Die we can all do.
Yield we shall never.
With a true Scottish heart
We'll charge together.

Come fill up my cup, come fill up my can,
Come saddle my horse and call up my man.
Come open your gates and let me gae free,
I dourna stay longer in bonny Dundee.

With Best Wishes to Nurse Goodban

Jock Whigham

In Remembrance of Nurse Goodban who departed from BRC Hospital Netley

2nd July 1918.

RIP
(**R**eturn **I**f **P**ossible)

Sgt Pittaway

CHAPTER THREE

ILFRACOMBE RED CROSS HOSPITAL

Nurse Goodban was in Ilfracombe on two occasions. From October 1914 until March 1915 she was at the Westwell Hospital and from October 1918 until January 31st 1919, when she left the Red Cross, she was at the Ilfracombe VA Hospital.

Ilfracombe was Nurse Goodban's home town at the time. After the war she carried on nursing and living in Ilfracombe. She eventually passed away in the town in 1968 when she was ninety years of age. She never married.

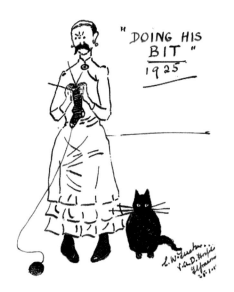

Message reads;

"DOING HIS BIT" 1925

E. W. Tucker VAD Hospital, Ilfracombe. 25/1/1919

(This patient/volunteer was not very optimistic – still expecting to be doing his duty in 1925!)

Lives of great men all remind us
We can make our lives sublime,
And departing leave behind us
Footprints on the sands of time.

27th January 1919
B*G Hayes*
CQMS

WHAT COUNTS

The day's work counts;
It isn't much
The gain of those few painful hours:
But be content if there is shown
Some product of those sacred powers
Which guide each mind, uphold each hand;
Strive with the best at your command –
The day's work counts.

29th January 1919
Sapper J Austin MM**
25th Division Signal Corps

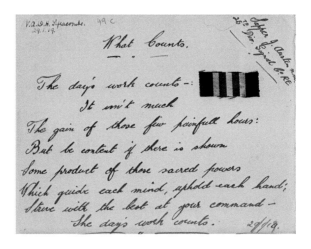

**This soldier is the only one to have indicated that he had been awarded a medal for bravery (Military Medal). I am sure other, more modest patients, were similarly decorated.

Many thanks to Nurse Goodban for all her kindness and the good and careful treatment in getting me so well. 30th January 1919

Best of wishes

Gunner W Braund
R.F.A.

There were several patients at Ilfracombe RCH that simply wrote their names:-

Private Fred Yeo 41247
East Lancs Regt
40 Division

Able Seaman Parsons, AFH
Royal Navy

Private S Baddick
1st Devons

(31st January 1919)

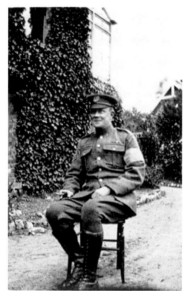
Sergeant House (?) Ilfracombe Hospital

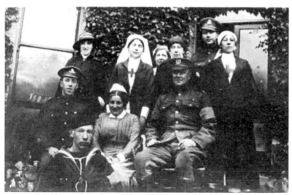
Patients and staff at Ilfracombe Hospital

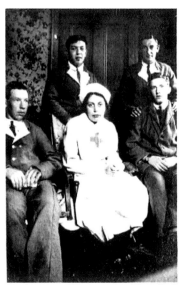

Patients at Ilfracombe Hospital

The story often repeated is that a sheet of paper divided into eight segments (see next), was routinely passed around the trauma ward and the incumbents were asked to fill in their details. Anyone correctly filling in the form was considered compos mentis and returned to duty. This may explain why the three listed waited until the war was over before completing the form!

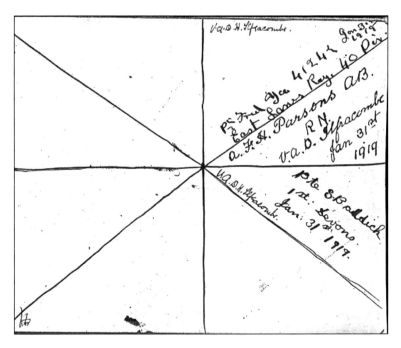

Men who signed paper are;

Private Fred Yeo 41247 East Lancs Regiment
Able Seaman A. F. H. Parsons, Royal Navy
Private E. Baddick, 1st Devons

31st January 1919

Private Ivor Davies
14 Royal Welsh Fusiliers
Wrexham N. Wales

Private W H Lee 73759
3rd Royal Welsh Fusiliers
Southport

Driver J* Gammon
C Battery
245 Brigade
R.F.A.

Driver C H Pearce
R.E. Signals
58th Division

Private C S* Wilson
4th Battalion
Devonshire Regiment

Lance Corporal Lawler
52nd (G) Battalion
Devonshire Regiment

21st February 1919

The fact that these men were still in hospital three months after the war ended, and obviously many months since they were in action, demonstrates the severity of their injuries. The cartoon of the elderly gentleman still "doing his bit" in 1925 gives an indication of how one particular person thought the treatment was going!

APPENDIX

Name	Rank	Number	Regiment	Hospital		Type of entry	Where/when wounded
Aitkin, Peter	Private	587	8th Brigade, Australian Forces	Netley	Photo	Poem	No details
Andrews, B.	Private		9th Essex Regiment	Netley			03/07/1916
Ardern, W.	Private		Lancashire Fusiliers	Barnstaple		Drawing	Messines - 7/06/1917
Armstrong, R.	Private		1st Royal Inniskillen Fusiliers	Barnstaple			Dardanelles - 1915 - Dysentary
Ashley, W.	Rifleman		The Rifle Brigade	Barnstaple			Trench fever - 1916
Austin, J. (Military Medal)	Sapper		26th Div Sigs - Royal Engineers	Ilfracombe	Photo	Poem and ribbon from medal.	No details
Baddick, S.	Private		1st Devonshire Regiment	Ilfracombe			No details
Bainbridge, R.	Private		22nd Durham Light Infantry	Netley	Photo	Poem	Delville Wood - Ardennes - 28/10/1916
Becker,	Gunner		121st Siege Battery R.G.A.	Netley	Photo	Poem	No details
Bennett, A.C.	Corporal		1/5th Gloucesters	Barnstaple			No details
Benson, J.J.	Private		2nd Bedford Regiment	Barnstaple		Poem	11/07/1916
Bentley, T.	Private		7th Notts and Derbys	Barnstaple		Poem	No details
Binns, A.H.	Private		1/6th West Yorkshire Regiment	Netley	Photo		No details
Borthwick, D.	Sapper		Royal Engineers - Telegraphs	Netley			No details
Braund, W.	Gunner		Royal Field Artillery	Ilfracombe	Photo		No details
Brewster, Albert	Gunner		D/5 Battery, Royal Field Artillery	Barnstaple	Photo	Poem	Ypres-Sept 1917
Browne, Gordon A.	Private		1/5 Norfolk Regiment	Barnstaple			Dardanelles - 13/08/1915
Brumbill	Private		1/1st Hereford Regiment	Barnstaple			No details
Bullock, W.	Private		Machine Gun Corps	Netley			Somme - 25/07/1916
Burn, R.M.	Corporal		Kings Own Yorks Lt Infantry	Barnstaple	Photo	Poem	No details
Burridge, L*	Sergeant		Irish Guards	Netley			No details
Butler, H	Private		3rd Dragoon Guards (Att. Buffs)	Barnstaple		Drawing	Vermelles - 1915 - Left shoulder, right leg
Chapman, A.F.	Trooper		Middlesex Hussars	Barnstaple			Dardanelles - 21/08/1915
Clark, (F)*	Private	291614	2/7 Devon Regiment	Barnstaple	Photo	Drawing-Best Medicine	No details
Clee, G.F.	Private		1 Bucks Battalion	Barnstaple	Slough	Drawing - Lady with chocolates	No details
Cook, L.	Private	948	2nd Queens RWS	Barnstaple			25/09/1915 & 1/07/1916
Davies, Thomas Ivor	Private		14th Royal Welsh Fusiliers	Ilfracombe			No details
Dudley, F.	Rifleman		The Rifle Brigade	Barnstaple		Poem	No details
Dudley, J.T.	Private		6th Notts and Derby	Netley			France - 1/07/1916
Durkins*, N.	Private		Loyal North Lancashires	Netley		Poem	Gallipoli and Mesopotania
Ellwood, Victor	Private		Duke of Wellingtons	Barnstaple	Photo		Dardanelles -1915
Elsworth, B.	Private	44019	9th Kings Own Yorks Light Inftry	Barnstaple		Drawing	No details
Elsworth, H	?		?	Barnstaple		Drawing-Yacht	Wounded 23/07/1916
E-------, H	Private	17491	75 Machine Gun Corps	Barnstaple			No details
Ferguson, Thomas (Jock)	Rifleman	2202	Scottish Rifles (Cameronians)	Barnstaple	Photo		Dardenelles - 28/06/1915
Fielder, H.	Rifleman		18th London Regt (London Irish)	Barnstaple		Drawing - Sailor boy and girlfriend	Ypres
Foot, Bert R.	Private		7th London Regiment	Netley			No details
Forbes* J	Private		1st Kensington Battalion	Barnstaple		Poem	Hebuterne - Somme 16/06/1916
Gallagher, S.J.	Corporal		9th Batt. Tyneside Scottish	Netley			Ypres - Wounded April, Gassed July 1916+H84
Gammon, J*	Driver		C Battery, 245 Brigade RFA	Ilfracombe			No details
Gauthier, H	Private	416379	22nd French Canadian Battalion	Netley		In French	No details
Gee, H.	Private	5830	13th Manchester Regiment	Netley	Photo	Poem	Macedonia-Trench foot-23/10/1916
Gregory, R.J.	Private		8th Devonshire Regiment	Barnstaple		Drawing and poem	Fricourt -Somme - 1/07/1916
Hamilton, J	Corporal		1st Battalion Black Watch	Barnstaple			Loos - Big Push - Right arm
Harris-James, A.O.	Rifleman		1st Queen's Westminster Rifles	Netley			Levanti - 23/01/1917
Hayes* B*G	CQMS		?	Ilfracombe		Poem	No details
Haynes*, S.E.	Rifleman		The Rifle Brigade	Ilfracombe		Poem	Big Push - 1916 - Gassed
Haylett, H.	Private		1/5 Norfolk	Barnstaple			Dardanelles - Dysentary and Neuralgia

Name	Rank		Regiment				
rst, F.	Corporal		10th Batt Yorksand Lancs Regt	Barnstaple		Quotation	Tricourt - 7/07/1916
orsham, H.	?		?	Netley	Guernsey		No details
ouse, H.	Lance Corporal		12th Middlesex Regiment	Netley			Somme - 14/07/1916 - Left leg
ughes, T.G*.	Corporal		Coldstream Guards	Netley	Photo		No details
hnson, M.	Lance Corporal		2nd Royal Irish Regiment	Barnstaple		Poem	Messines - 7/06/1917
pling, J.V.	Sapper	9453	Australian Engineers	Netley		Drawing - Young lady	No details
aminski, E.A.	Lance Corporal		8th Canadian Infantry Battalion	Netley			Somme Push -26/09/1916
ay, H	?		12th Hampshire Regiment	Netley		Drawing - Arab gentleman	Salonica
ermode, G.N.	Private		?	Barnstaple	Photo		No details
ghtley, T.R.	?		Royal Field Artillery	Barnstaple		Poem	No details
lgour, J	Lance Corporal		9th Black Watch	Barnstaple			Loos - 25/09/1915
obb, J. W.	Lance Corporal		1st QVR, 9th London Regiment	Barnstaple			No details
ne, C.J.	Sapper		Royal Engineers- Signals	Netley		Quotation	No details
wler,	Lance Corporal		52nd Batt. Devonshire Regiment	Ilfracombe	Photo		No details
e, W.H.	Private	73759	3rd Royal Welsh Fusiliers	Ilfracombe	Photo/Southport		No details
ster*, G.	Private		16th West Yorkshire	Barnstaple		Poem	No details
nd, H.	Driver	32816	64th Battery, Royal Field Artillery	Netley			No details
aybin, A.	Private		7th battalion East Surrey	Barnstaple		Poem	No details
c Conaghy, J.	Driver		Royal Field Artillery	Barnstaple	Photo	Drawing - Baby in high chair	No details
illard, C.	Private		9th East Surreys	Barnstaple		Poem	01/06/1916
orley, Joe	Private		?	Barnstaple	Photo		No details
urdoch, C.	Private		1/6* Gordons	Netley		Drawing - Sweetheart	Wounded - 17/7, 25/9/15, & 13/3/16
ash, E.F.	Sergeant		1st Gloucestershire Regiment	Barnstaple			Loos - 24/09/1915 -
cholson, J.	Lance Corporal		?	Netley			No details
arsons, A.F.H.	Able Seaman		Royal Navy	Ilfracombe			No details
earce, C.H.	Driver		58th Div. Royal Engineer - Signals	Ilfracombe			No details
illips, F.C.	Rifleman		1st Queen's Westminster Rifles	Barnstaple		Quotation	Gommecourt - 1/07/1916
per	Able Seaman		Royal Navy	Ilfracombe	Photo		No details
etrovski, P.W.	Private		15th Canadian Infantry Battalion	Netley			Somme Push - 26/09/1916
ttaway, M.G.	Sergeant		?	Netley	Photo		No details
eddy, T.	Private		9th Devonshire Regiment	Netley		Short verse	Somme - 01/07/1916
uirke* P.J.	Lance Corporal		1st Royal Dublin Fusiliers	Barnstaple		Short verse	No details
ackham,	Sapper		Royal Engineers	N etley		Poem	No details
eid, F.H.	Private		2nd Middlesex Regiment	Barnstaple		Epic Poem	Poiziers - 1/07/1916-Shoulder/thigh
ess, T.	Lance Corporal	145	6th RW Kent Regiment	Barnstaple			Vermelles?
obbins, Vincent E.	Rifleman		1st Queen Victoria's Rifles				Gommecourt - Somme Push - 1/07/1916
obinson	?		?	Netley			No details
ock, F.	?		?	Netley		Poem	No details
dler, S.C.	Private		Machine Gun Corps	Barnstaple	Welsh	Quotation	Neuve Chapelle 19/08/1916
mwell, G.E.	Private		1st Royal Fusiliers	Barnstaple	Photo		Hooge? France - 6/7/1915 - Right arm
ndiford,	Corporal		154 Brigade R.F.A.	Barnstaple		Drawing - boy in bath	France 1916
llers, R.C.	Private		10th Canadian Infantry	Netley		Prose	Somme - 26/09/1916 - L. knee & arms
arp, C	Rifleman		1/6th London Regiment	Netley		Drawings - Flapper & Vicar	No details
ayler*, D.	Private		11th Royal Fusiliers	Netley			France - 23/01/1916
inner, A.J.	Sergeant		1st Battalion Rifle Brigade	Netley		Poem	No details
ack, H.	Private		16th Queen's Regiment	Netley		Poem	No details
lly, J*	Corporal		2nd Borderers	Barnstaple	Photo		Givenchy - 10/10/15 - Right arm
afford, A.G.	Private	724	5th Australian Mach.Gun Batt.	Netley	Photo		No details
anley, F.	Lance Corporal		94th Fld Co, Royal Engineers	Barnstaple		Poem	No details

Name	Rank	Number	Regiment	Location		Photo	Drawing/Poem	Details
Steel, John	Lance Corporal		Royal Scots Fusiliers	Barnstaple	Beith/Ayrshire		Poem	No details
Sutton*, A.	Gunner		66th S.Battery R.G.A.	Netley			Poem	Somme - 10/10/1916
Sutton, G.	Lance Corporal		1/5th North Staffs Regiment	Barnstaple			Poem	18/08/1915 & 1/07/1916
Taylor, Frank	Private	15919	2nd Dorsets, 6 Poona Division	Netley			Poem	Mesopotania
Thomas, David Anthony	Sergeant		R.H.A.	Barnstaple		Photo	Poem	No details
Thomas, F*	Private		9th Welsh Regiment	Barnstaple				France - 25/09/1915 - Face
Tiptod*, R.	Lance Corporal		1/5 Norfolks	Barnstaple		Photo	Drawing - Lady in hat	No details
Travers, E.			6th (Inniskillen?) Dragoons	Netley				No details
Truss, P.J.	Private	2073162	Infantry - A.S.C.	Netley				No details
Tucker, E.W.	?		?	Ilfracombe			Drawing - Old man knitting	No details
Venables, H.	Trooper		6th Inniskillen Dragoons	Barnstaple		Photo		No details
Walker, C.	Bombadier		?	Netley				No details
Walker, E.	Gunner		?	Netley				No details
Walker, J.	C.Q.M.Sergeant		11th Battalion East Lancs Regt	Barnstaple		Photo	Drawing - nurse	No details
Walsh, A.	Private		Scottish Highlanders	Barnstaple		Photo	Drawing- German soldier	No details
Wells, Louis J.	?		?	Barnstaple				Gommecourt - 1/07/1916
Whigham, (Jock)	?		?	Netley			Poem	No details
Wilson, C.R.*	Private		4th Battalion Worcestershires	Ilfracombe				No details
Wiseman, George	?		M.T. A.S.C.	Barnstaple				Hebatune - 20/06/1916
Yeo, Fred	Private	41247	40th Div. East Lancs Regiment	Ilfracombe				No details